SHEENA LEIGH

10 Minute Workouts for Couch Potatoes

Your simple, straightforward guide to getting moving at home!

Contents

1

Disclaimer

Please note that the information contained in this book is written for educational and entertainment purposes only. I have used all efforts to present accurate, reliable and up-to-date information. This book is not to be used for medical diagnosis or treatment recommendation. I am not a medical or healthcare professional. Always talk to your healthcare provider if you have any questions concerning your health. I am not engaging in rendering any medical or professional advice. I am not liable for any action a reader takes upon reading this information.

2

Introduction

Welcome to 10 Minute Workouts for Couch Potatoes! My name is Sheena Leigh and I am so excited to be writing this book for you! Today I am an avid mover, maybe even a workout junkie, but I wasn't always. Taking small steps, learning to get up, get moving and understanding that doing just a little every day really does add up has literally saved my life and I want to share this life hack with you!

There was a time in my 20's when I was the BIGGEST couch potato! I was the absolute queen of reading, watching TV, sitting at the kitchen table gabbing or playing cards or board games... I was an Indoor Kid. I had just left college and was working the first of my many serving jobs to come. I was a little certain of where I wanted to go in life... and I was also trying out a lot of paths and feeling into what kind of life I was going to build. I was also slamming head first into the humbling life lesson of Paying Back Student Debt while learning to Life (*cue dramatic daunting music)! So things were strange and busy to say the least! When I'd get home all I would want is to sink into the couch and let the day melt away. Alone, with loved ones, with food, with a good book and tea, with my cat, with my dog or both! However and in whatever way, I was a couch potato and I loved it!

And I got so depressed.

For me it was depression. For you and others the signs that we may not be engaged with our lives in the best way we could be will vary. You know. You know why you picked out this book. You know what keeps you in the story in your head that you can't get up and move a little today. Or maybe that life is stuck. That today is a good day to relax, a rest day. Like the day before, and the day before that... and the day before that. I know, I've been there. I was right there on that couch, tucked into whatever narrative kept me safe and the same. Kept me right where I Knew What Would Happen. And I was bored. So bored! I felt stagnant. Do you know what I mean?

Well, one day, I don't know why, one day I got up. I just couldn't stay glued to my couch and I decided to get up and get Started and do SOMETHING. I just wanted to feel my heart beat and my temperature rise and feel my breath in my lungs.

I did jumping jacks.

I felt so silly! There I was doing jumping jacks in my living room at 11:30pm on a Wednesday. I was supposed to be an adult now who knew about Stuff. But I didn't know what to do so I jumped and swung my arms until I was laughing and giggling and having a whole lot of fun! After a few minutes I stopped and stood and felt my heart and my lungs and the beginnings of a sheen of sweat on my forehead. I felt better. I felt good. I sat back down and finished the last few pages of the chapter of my book and was smiling a bit as I went to bed. I slept better than I had in forever. And I was hooked! How could so little, such a silly little piece of movement have such a big impact?

For me I went on a mission, a deep dive into health and wellness modalities. I faced my fear of inverting and finally discovered yoga, which felt like coming home. I trained in Ashtanga, Vinyasa and Iyengar styles. I also became a nationally certified personal trainer and was coaching clients in working out, wellness and nutrition. I bridged all this self-sought education with my decades of training as a dancer and circus performer over the years and began to understand the amazing connection between movement and my overall well being.

That is what I hope to give to you in these pages!

This book isn't necessarily one you will sit down and read cover to cover. My hope is that this book is a go-to reference for you. One where you see the reminder on your phone to get up and move, maybe you sigh, doubt and distraction fighting you, and you grab this book, open to a workout and get started!

So, let's get into it!

3

What to Expect

In this book you are getting a straightforward guide to getting moving at home. We will go over a bit about why we are going to move in these ways, talk about our mental approach, how long to move, what exactly to do and easy lifestyle habits you can begin to enact in your everyday life to feel better. We cover warming up, cooling down, stretching, tips on practicing good form, getting moving with what you have at home, and of course, the workouts! Straightforward and simple. Just as getting started on your fitness journey should be. You know what they say, KISS... keep it simple silly!

4

Accountability

I am writing this book as an able-bodied human who does not navigate disability personally. I recognize this book is not written with disabled bodies in mind. I am inexperienced in this area and will not only do my best here to offer a helpful approach to continuing to use this book w/ a disability, but I will also recognize and take this opportunity to see where I can improve as a teacher and a work out enthusiast.

If you are a person living with a disability and you are here to get moving, let's do just that! As we proceed through these first sections and chapters I speak into utilizing what we have and meeting ourselves where we are. That is what I believe I can offer to you as well. What we are really trying to accomplish here is getting our heart rates up a bit, warming up our body temperature and experiencing the endorphins we get from doing those things. Those effects can be created in many, many ways so work with what you have. Move the parts and places you safely can. Choose a range and speed that works for you, that gets you to feel your heart and raise your temperature in some way.* We will discuss how focused and intentional breathing can be your workout for the day. We will discuss mindfulness and how 10 minutes a day can produce beautiful benefits for our overall health. Working with moving only a single limb, in small motions, from a seated position, or only one exercise for a few minutes... there is no wrong. There is only what serves.

Wherever you are, work within your reasonable limits. I'll say this a few times. KISS. Keep It Simple Silly! You are here reading this book and taking a step towards yourself and your health. That is exactly where we all need to be and the best place to make the best next decision for ourselves. I'm glad you're here!

In whatever way you can, let's get moving!

Please see the Disclaimer at the beginning of this book.

5

Why Body Weight Workouts

The first concept to understand is that small steps add up to big results. Experts and top trainers across the industry agree that body weight exercises serve as a key foundation to well-rounded overall health. Body weight exercise is strength training that uses your own body to provide resistance. Simple as that. Body weight workouts are any series of movements where you use only your own body to provide the resistance. Most people have done body weight exercises and just may not have realized it. Some common examples of body weight exercises are Push Ups, Planks, Squats, Lunges and Crunches.

Body weight exercise builds strength, balance, cardio, flexibility and mobility all at the same time. That means we couch potatoes can rest assured knowing we are getting as much impact from each bit of effort we exude. Very often these workouts end up being full body because you are using your own body as your weight set. This engages multiple muscles at the same time as well as major muscles repeatedly in different ways, working the muscles to fatigue quicker and more efficiently. This is fantastic because it makes the entire body work to stabilize and support itself also. These compound movements all add up to building more overall strength. The tendons and ligaments engage and stretch, broadening your range of flexibility while strengthening the supportive elements our body relies on for being mobile as well as balancing. With multiple systems working at the same time you also trigger your heart to pump faster and at differing and changing tempos, training your cardiovascular system.

Using your body as your gym means your workouts are endlessly adjustable. If you are brand new to working out a simple 10 minute body weight series is plenty to get your whole body started on this journey with you. If you already do a little cardio at the gym then adding a few body weight exercises after as a pre-cool down can have a massive effect on your results. Adjusting the intensity of your workout on any given day is a simple matter of adjusting your number of repetitions, tempo or the form of your movements. So straightforward you can truly do these exercises almost anywhere; in your living room, in a hotel room, at a park, in your office, at the gym... anywhere there is space to move. Also and maybe most importantly, it's free! You don't need anything other than your own Self to get a full body workout in and reap all its benefits. Body weight exercises are accessible to everyone and support anyone at any stage of their fitness journey. For us couch potatoes this is everything!!

You'll find that body weight workouts are generally not too different from each other and that is a good thing. What I mean is, it's a lot of the same moves in different arrangements or done in different ways and to different rhythms. The reason for this is simple, since we are using our body as the gym we are always working within our human range of motion. That gives all our movements a space and range they stay in. This works to our advantage for two reasons. One: we repeat similar movements over and over again, building consistency and muscle memory. Consistency builds muscle over time (small steps ;) and repetition builds knowledge, confidence and surety. When we know what we are doing we are free to engage with that thing much more. Simplifying movement in this way helps make it more accessible. Two: we are most often working within our usable frame of movement. Meaning the work we are putting in is building muscles we really use everyday, not ones we can only really isolate on a machine at the gym. Our body is a complex system, everything relies on everything else to some degree. We are never using just one muscle to accomplish a task, muscles are always working with a team of other muscles, tendons, ligaments, tissues and bones to move your arm up and down. Machines and super specialized exercises are great for isolating and working on specific areas and muscles. There is a place for that training, in sports and specialist movers for example, but for a couch potato getting up to simply move for 10 minutes a day, we don't need all that and actually benefit more from compound movements that mimic our everyday activities. Straightforward, effective and simple is the name of that game!

A 2017 study in the Journal of Osteopathic Medicine showed that exercise significantly decreased perceived stress and improved physical, mental and emotional health in medical students. The data is pretty unanimous across the board that incorporating any kind of movement into your time eases not only the body but the mind and our emotional states. We know that exercise releases mood-boosting endorphins into our brains and that chemical is the best high any of us can chase! Moving our body can help reduce anxiety symptoms, calm social anxieties and generally ground us in our sense of Self. The mix of good brain chemicals and improved sleep supports us in feeling better and generally having a more open and positive outlook on our lives. Whether its walking, jogging, a bike ride, a sport, gardening, a short yoga flow or just a few situps and pushups to start your day, finding something you enjoy and doing a little bit of that often adds up to a whole lot of healthy steps.

6

Mindset

Ok, now we are going to take this one step deeper. Let's be honest here, you picked up this book for a reason. Heck, I was inspired to write this book for a reason! We all generally seek information, support and reassurance when we know we need a change in some way in our lives.

That is your mindset shifting.

And that's possibly the most important piece in this whole Getting Moving puzzle! I want to acknowledge and celebrate you for being here and being open to changing your mind. There is a famous saying "whether you think you can or think you can't, you're right." What we tell ourselves about ourselves is so deeply important to how we see ourselves. And how we see ourselves is how we show up in the world, 100% of the time. Being open to changing our habits, to seeing ourselves in a new light is truly the most important step in any fitness journey. Just acknowledging that improvement is possible is a foundational first step!

This book is absolutely written to help support anyone in revising their mental perspective. One key way to do this is exactly what we have been focusing on: 'moving' over 'exercising'. Our bodies are designed for movement so by simply asking ourselves what gets us up and moving is a perfect place to start. And whatever ideas pop up are great! Because they are inspiring to You and therefore are exactly what you need. Taking the stairs instead of the elevator, having a 5 minute dance break in your office or opening up to a 10 minute workout in this book and getting your heart pumping while catching up on that tv series are all perfect ways to just get up and get moving! As long as you're having fun and moving your body, you're doing it right!

7

Tools That Help

Breath work

Breath work refers to deep, diaphragmatic or belly breathing. Research suggests augmenting our breath in these ways may trigger relaxation responses in the body. From long and slow to fast and deep, the term Breath work encompasses a range of breathing exercises designed to enhance overall and physical health. We know that by focusing on our breath and breathing in these patterns we shift our body's chemistry, clean and oxygenate our blood, and participate actively in shifting our mindset. We can clear old emotions or get incredibly present, both help support us in feeling what we and our bodies want and need.

Types of Breath work to be curious about:

- Holotropic
- Pyramid Breath
- Pranayama
- Rebirthing

- Alternate nostril breathing
- Box breathing

...to name a few.

Meditation

Mediation is different in that it focuses on the mind, or maybe getting out of the mind. The Miriam Webster definition of mediation is to engage in contemplation or reflection. Simply put, meditation is intentionally spending time with ourselves, focusing, becoming aware of our thoughts, practicing staying present and letting our thoughts go. It teaches us compassion and empathy, first for ourselves and then for others. We learn to listen to ourselves, really listen, and hold ourselves in our sincerest Truth. From that place of honesty within ourselves we understand and get to practice forgiveness and acceptance. This puts us in the driver's seat and supports us in making the choices we really want to make or at least the ones that may be harder to make at first.

Benefits of Meditating:

- Feel calmer overall
- Clear-headedness
- More comfortable with their own minds
- Increased patience
- Increased creativity
- Lower resting heart rates

- Lowered stress
- Better success managing their stress
- Supported anxiety management
- Reduction in chronic pain
- Enhanced willpower
- Better sleep.

All of these benefits together support us in making the seemingly simple choices everyday to create the life we want.

We can't lie to ourselves, not really. When we make the space and time to feel our feelings (intentionally breathing) and witness our thoughts (focused quiet time with ourselves) we learn we have all the information we need to care best for ourselves and do what needs to be done. These tools can be utilized for as little as 10 minutes a day almost anywhere, especially from the comfort of your couch, and can provide exponential benefits for us physically, mentally and emotionally.

8

What 10 Minutes A Day Can Do

Studies show that in as little as 10 minutes a day a session of moderate to vigorous activity can provide a shocking amount of benefits. It's been found that short bursts of intense exercise before meals actually help control blood sugar better than a 30 minute workout does. This can allow for more control of blood sugar levels and may lower risk of diabetes. Just by getting the heart pumping for three minutes there is improved oxygen absorption supports overall endurance and cardiovascular stamina. There is even research showing that 10 minutes of high intensity interval training can give the same benefits as a 45 minute jog!

We have already discussed how such a short amount of time shifts our mood, concentration and mindset. Shorter sessions provide quite a lot of flexibility in type and style of movement. Keeping things interesting with variety helps support us in coming back and choosing to move again. Shorter workouts are also more easily achievable which activates our reward center in the brain supporting us repeating that rewarded action... which is moving our body again. And we all know another well-known phrase "consistency is king!" Little steps often will always get us where we want to go. Grand large steps sometimes might, but very often they fall short of actually getting us to wherever we need to be. Consistency and repetition become so much easier when we are only dedicating 10 minutes a day!

9

What You'll Need

Calling back to our discussion earlier about the benefits of body weight exercises, what is absolutely great about body weight workouts is that you don't need anything to get moving! With that said, there are many options available around our homes everyday to help us elevate our movement time, either in intensity or fun. There are also important options available to make us feel safe. We will cover both.

Space

First and foremost we need some space! One of the things a gym offers is a dedicated Place where movement happens. That can exist in our home too! We don't need much space, again, body weight exercises mean we are usually working within a reasonable average range of our own motion. If you can lay a yoga mat down and swing your arms around your sides, you have enough space to move your body.

I began by leaving my yoga mat rolled up next to my couch. It was a not so subtle reminder to myself that I truly want to move more. Once I had laid out my mat I could technically just roll around on it and stretch a bit and that was technically moving my body for the day. And I was right. Which felt great every single time. And as I laid there rolling around on the ground stretching some life back into my limbs and feeling my heart beat a little quicker in my chest, absolutely pleased with myself, I was only too happy to continue feeling better! And I'd roll my way into some version of stretching or yoga or transitioning to standing and there I was... a few minutes into moving. Whatever I chose to do from then on, I had already won. Simply by giving myself the space, or sometimes referred to as permission ;) to move.

Equipment

There are certain tools you will find in every gym and most workouts are based around utilizing these tools. With many of our workouts in this book we are working in the other direction. We are beginning with everyday functional movements and adding intensity to them through body positioning, repetition and engagement. You will find that most of these tools are 'built in" to the body weight exercise segments in this book. Where a workout may offer a level-up by adding some additional weight to our body or limbs there are almost always perfect substitutions within arms reach! Let's cover some.

<u>*Equipment You May Want and At-Home Alternatives*</u>

Yoga Mat ~ A towel, the floor, literally nothing

Dumbbells ~ Milk Jugs, Soup Cans, Water Bottle, anything with some weight that is easy to grip, a little goes a long way.

Resistance Bands ~ Old pantyhose or tights, anything stretchy you can hold onto.

Step Bench ~ Step Stools can work, Stable Chairs. Also substitute a hop or jumping in place of stepping up.

Jump Rope ~ Anything long, slender and swingable thing will do!

Stability Ball ~ Not as necessary as you may think! Try engaging in your abdominal work on the floor more precisely. For challenging balance try closing your eyes or adjusting your angle on a piece of furniture or a wall. For challenging abdominal work try supporting just your upper or lower spine on the seat of a chair with a towel for comfort.

Bench ~ Most things done on a bench are just as effective as when they are done on the floor. If you have 2 matching dining room or folding chairs, setting them side by side can give you some options as well. Engage precisely and increase your reps or weight.

Dip/Push Up Bar ~ Not necessary! Use the couch!

Weighted Vest ~ Try carrying something weighted, a few pounds is all you need; a bag of rice or dry beans on each shoulder.

Kettlebells, Sand Bags, etc. ~ See Dumbells

Machines and Large Equipment ~ Don't need em!!

Remember when it comes to getting moving, when in doubt, Keep It Simple Silly!

Things You May Actually Want Close By

Water
A Towel
Music
Timer or Clock
A fan
Notebook or Dry Erase board to track
A Foam Roller for recovering after in front of the couch

Remember to use whatever you have at your disposal. Balance a hand on the cat tree for support. Use the couch!! Do tricep dips on it, lean on the back for angled push ups. Heck, jump on it like a trampoline (if that's safe) and it gets you moving and smiling like a kid! Remember one of the best benefits of moving at home is that you get to do whatever you want and need to support yourself in getting moving.

10

The Warm Ups

This is it! This is where we get moving! If you have skipped ahead to this spot, wonderful! You've come to the right place! We begin any movement session with a little warming up before really getting into it. Why? Because we want to get our blood moving, raise the temperature in our body a bit and introduce the idea of moving to our muscles. You can get fancy and have the movements you use in your warm up mimic the exercises you plan to do to specifically warm up those muscle groups. For our purposes we just want to engage in any light activity that raises our heartbeat and gets us to start to sweat for 3–5 minutes.

Easy Mobility Warm Up

- 2 minutes Marching in Place

Option for hands on hips or arms swinging naturally by sides

• 60 seconds alternating Heel Digs in front of you.

Option to extend arms out to sides or in front and hold

• 30 seconds alternating Knee Lifts

Option to touch opposite hand to knee as lifting

• 10 Shoulder Rolls each direction

Option to go back to Heel Digs or stand still

• 15 Mini Squats, halfway down and up

Option for arms to bicep curl as you lower and straighten as you do

One and Done Warm Ups

This is a list of easy to moderately active things you can do to warm up as opposed to a series of moves. Do any of them for at least 3 minutes, up to 10. Ps. If you do 10 minutes of any of these that counts as moving your body today!

1. Brisk Walk
2. Jog
3. Jumping Jacks
4. Dance to Your Favorite Song
5. Climb Your Stairs
6. Plank

7. Jump Rope
8. Engaged Stretching
9. Sun Salutation A
10. Moon Salutation

Joint Mobility Warm Up

· Hip Circles

Stand centered on two feet, hands on your hips and slowly start to draw circles with your hips. Forward, side, back, side. Whichever direction you start with, circle a few times and then switch directions.

· Hip Swings

Stand on one leg, use the couch for support, and gently swing the free leg in circles to the side. Play with the size of your circles and tempo for a few rotations, then switch sides and repeat.

· Arm Circles

Stand comfortably between two feet, arms stretched horizontal out to the sides, palms facing down. Begin tracing circles one way for a few rotations, then go the other way.

· Arm Swings

Stand comfortably between two feet, arms stretched forward, horizontal, palms facing down. Take a step forward and swing your arms in unison to the right so your left arm is in front of your chest and fingers point to the right. Keep your body and head neutral facing forward; move only at the shoulders. Take another step forward and swing the arms to the left so your right arm is in front of your chest and your fingers point to the left. Take a few steps forward. Bonus Challenge; take a few steps back.

- Standing Marches

Stand comfortably between two parallel feet, arms loose at your sides. Step with your left foot and raise your right knee in a march. Then repeat as you lower the right foot, lift the left knee in a march. Let the arms swing naturally as you do this. Lift the knees higher or change the tempo as needed.

- Stepping Over Walk

Again, start standing comfortably between two parallel feet, hands on your hips. Lift your right foot and deeply flex your toes towards you. Step down on your heel and slowly roll through each part of your foot as you complete your step. Bonus challenge, also let your knee bend as you lower your foot. Then straighten your right leg as you lift the left foot, super flex the left toes towards you as you rise up onto the toes of the right foot beneath you. Slowly step deeply down through the left heel, rolling through each part of your left foot as you complete the step. Bonus Challenge; continue to bend the knee as you lower and rise up onto the ball of each foot as you walk slowly forward a few steps. Extra Bonus Challenge; walk a few steps backwards the same way.

- Walking Twisted Lunges

Start standing comfortably between two parallel feet, arms loose at your sides. Take an exaggerated step forward, rolling through your foot to plant it solidly beneath your leg. Then bend both knees equally to lower into a lunge. Keep your forward knee over the ankle and your back knee from touching the ground. Let the arms naturally swing around you gently twisting in your spine. Press your front foot off the ground to push back to standing. Repeat on the other side a few times til you feel your heart beating.

4.5 Minute Warm Up

1. 30 Seconds; Toe Touches, reach out one leg in front of you and touch your toe to the ground then step the foot back next to your other one. Repeat with your other foot, setting a tempo and moving briskly.

2. 30 Seconds; Stand with your feet wider than your hips. Step on one foot, let your body twist naturally to that side and your arms reach wide open at shoulder level while you stretch the opposite leg straight and touch the toe. Then repeat on your other foot, stepping and letting the body naturally twist. The arms follow along, coming into the center between steps and opening it whichever side when you step. Keep your tempo.

3. 30 Seconds; Keep stepping side to side but keep your torso forward. Now instead of touching alternating toes begin bending alternating knees back behind you. Pull your elbows behind you with each bend of the knee and reach forward as you step. Try to not let your tempo falter.

4. 30 Seconds; Keep stepping side to side with your torso facing forward. Change your legs to lifting alternating knees up to the side

towards each armpit. Alternate touching opposite hands to each knee as you lift it. Try to maintain your tempo through the rest of your warm up.

5. 30 Seconds; Stand still, feet in a wide stance, arms stretched out horizontally to your sides, like a star. As you inhale, bend forward and reach your right fingers to your left toes. It doesn't matter if you touch them, just that you aim in the direction of your toes. Exhale as you straighten back up arms reaching back out wide. Repeat on the other side. Inhale reaches left fingers to right toes, exhale engages your glutes as you straighten back up, arms reaching wide.

6. 30 Seconds; Non-Jumping Jumping Jacks. Exactly what they sound like. Do everything in a jumping jack except jump off the ground. Use alternating step touches to your sides instead.

7. 30 Seconds; Continue with your non jumping jacks but change the legs to alternating knee raises in front of you. Arms stay the same, swinging over head.

8. 30 Seconds; Step to the side, turn your torso to that side, reach your opposite arm up across your body at a diagonal as you reach your opposite leg straight, tapping the toe to your other side. Step on your other foot now (the toe you just tapped), turn your torso to that side as your opposite arm reaches up across your body at a diagonal as you reach you first leg straight to tap that toe. Continue stepping, twisting and reaching side to side.

9. 30 Seconds; Finally, face forward and step with alternating knee raises. This time pull alternating elbows towards the rising knee. Finish out with a strong tempo!

11

The Workouts

It's time to get moving! You've already moved for a few minutes in your warm up, hopefully your joints are feeling a little softer, your muscles are warm and loose and your heart is ready to get pumping!

Use this section as a reference guide. Mark your favorite sequences, flip back and forth, try a little of everything. Find the flavor of movement that, well, moves you! When we are having fun we are more likely to repeat that Thing over again. So have fun and remember, as long as you are moving your body and feeling good you are doing it right!

These circuits can be done 1-3 times through. You can also jump from one style to another, whatever keeps you inspired and moving for at least 10 minutes a day. Engage with each movement precisely to create more or less resistance. Feel free to add a small weight to your hands when available, but this isn't necessary.

Let's get moving!

Full Body, Body Weight

Body Weight 1

- Body Weight Squat - 15-25 Reps

Stand evenly between two feet, hip distance apart, arms down by your sides. Inhale as you bend both knees and reach your hips back behind you, keeping your knees over your toes as you lower down, creating a 90 degree angle with your legs. At the same time your arms bend at the elbow, bringing your hands either to your chest or straight out in front of you (or hold onto the couch for support). Exhale and press through your feet, engaging your leg muscles to stand up and drop your hands back down by your sides. Repeat.

- Push Ups - 10-15 Reps

Get down on the floor into a push up position, either on your toes or on your knees. Place a towel or yoga mat under your knees for support if needed. You can also do these standing by leaning at an angle against a wall, a counter or the back of a couch.

Place your hands at least shoulders width apart, maybe wider. Pull your belly button in towards your spine. Inhale to bend at the elbows lowering your body down almost to the floor, then exhale and push back up to your starting position. Repeat.

There are hundreds of ways to do a Push Up. Do what feels available to your body. If it hurts in a bad way, change something. Keep going!!

- Stepping Lunges - 10-15 Each Leg

Stand evenly between two feet, hip distance apart, hands on your waist. Inhale, taking an exaggerated step forward, rolling through your foot to plant it solidly beneath your leg. Then bend both knees equally to lower into a 90 degree lunge. Keep your forward knee over the ankle and your back knee from touching the ground. Press your front foot off the ground to push back to standing. Repeat.

- No Dumbbell Rows - 15-25 Reps

Stand evenly between two feet, hip distance apart. Pull your belly button in and lean forward with a straight back, about 45 degrees. Let your arms hang down towards the ground, hands in fists. Keeping your elbows close in towards your body, exhale and bend your elbows, pulling your fists to your ribs, resisting like you are pulling something heavy. Inhale to push your fists towards the ground like you are pushing something into the ground beneath you. Pull your belly button to your spine again and repeat.

- Plank - 15-60 Seconds

Get down on the floor into a push up position, either on your toes or on your knees. Place a towel or yoga mat under your knees for support if needed. Breathe steadily as you pull your belly button to your spine. Lengthen your spine, reaching your crown and heels away from each other. Close your lower ribs and re-engage your belly button to your spine. Through your heels, stretch your legs long and strong behind you. Drop your shoulders away from your ears, feeling your shoulder blades shift down your spine. Wrap your shoulder blades around the sides of your rib cage. Press the ground away from you through your arms, extending your reach. Re-engage your belly button to your spine. Re-read this paragraph until you reach your time goal.

- Double Jumping Jacks - 15-60 Seconds

Begin by doing regular jumping jacks, jumping both feet out wide while swinging your arms straight out to the sides and above your head, then jumping both feet back in underneath you as your arms swing back down to your sides again. Once you have this rhythm begin double jumping in both positions, keeping the arms where they are for the extra beat. Set a tempo and keep it up until you reach your time goal.

- Curtsy Squats - 10-15 Each Leg

Just like our first set of squats, stand evenly between two feet, hip distance apart, but hands on your hips. This time as you inhale and bend your knees you will step your right foot behind you and across to your left as much as you reasonably can, in a curtsy. Keep your left knee over your toes by reaching your hips back and keeping your chest lifted as you lower down, bend your right leg down to a 90 degree angle keeping your knee from touching the ground. Exhale and press through your left foot to stand back up, setting your right foot back in its original place. Repeat on the other side.

Body Weight 2

- Jumping Jacks - 15-60 Seconds

Jump both feet out wide while swinging your arms straight out to your sides and above your head, then jumping both feet back in underneath you as your arms swing back down to your sides again. Once you have this rhythm begin double jumping in both positions, keeping the arms where they are for the extra beat. Set a tempo and keep it until you reach your time goal.

- Pulsing Squat - 15-25 Reps

Stand evenly between two feet, hip distance apart, arms down by your sides. Take a short inhale as you bend both knees as you reach your hips back behind you, keeping your knees over your toes as you lower down, legs creating a 90 degree angle. At the same time your arms bend at the elbow, bringing your hands either to your chest or straight out in front of you (or hold onto the couch for support). Take another short inhale as you pulse the bend in your knees.

Fully exhale as you press through your feet to stand up, engaging your leg muscles as you do and dropping your hands back down by your sides. Repeat.

- Mountain Climbers - 15-60 Seconds

Start in your high plank position. Setting a tempo, pull your right knee in toward the center of your chest and then step it back to plank, then pull the left knee in and step it back. Keep alternating legs, engage your belly button to your spine, stabilizing your body parallel to the floor.

- Burpees - 15-25 Reps

Stand evenly between two feet, hip distance apart, arms down by your sides. Reach down to the ground. Place your hands on the floor under your shoulders and hop or step your feet back to a plank. Do a push up, either on your toes or by dropping your knees. Then hop or step your feet back up to your hands. Press through your feet to jump up, straightening your legs and reaching your arms overhead. Land softly then repeat, reaching your hands down to the ground.

- Reverse Lunges - 10-15 Each Leg

Stand evenly between two feet, hip distance apart, hands on your hips. Inhale to take an exaggerated step back behind you with your right leg, leaving your left foot rooted into the ground. Bend each leg, creating a 90-degree angle with your left leg and keeping your right knee from touching the ground. Exhale and push through your right foot, stepping back to your starting position. Repeat, alternating legs.

- Forearm Plank - 15-60 Seconds

Start in your plank position. Place a towel or yoga mat under your knees for support if needed. Place your forearms on the floor, parallel to each other or clasping hands, as long as your elbows are below your shoulders. Breathe steadily as you pull your belly button to your spine. Lengthen your spine, reaching your crown and heels away from each other. Close your lower ribs and re-engage your belly button to your spine. Through your heels, stretch your legs long and strong behind you. Drop your shoulders away from your ears, feeling your shoulder blades shift down your spine. Wrap your shoulder blades around the sides of your rib cage. Press your forearms into the ground. Re-engage your belly button to your spine. Re-read this paragraph until you reach your time goal.

- Hip Dips - 15-60 Seconds

Maintain your forearm plank position, engaging your abdominals. Drop your right hip down towards the floor, then bring it back up to neutral. Repeat with your left hip. Set a tempo and alternate hips until you reach your time goal.

Body Weight 3

• Jogging in Place - 15-60 Seconds

Begin by running easily in place, letting your arms swing naturally by your sides as they will. Focus on picking up your feet, breathing steadily, setting a tempo and maintaining it.

• Sumo Squats - 15-25 Reps

Stand with your feet set wide, toes turned out, arms fist to fist at your chest. Inhale as you bend both knees, keeping your chest lifted as you reach your bottom low behind you, guiding your knees over your toes as you lower down. Arms can stay at your chest or open to cactus arms as you squat. Exhale and press through your feet, engaging your leg muscles to stand up, bringing your hands to your chest again. Repeat.

• Leg Lifts - 10-15 Each Leg

Lay down on a mat, a towel or the floor. Pull your belly button down to your spine and flatten your lower back on the floor. Extend your arms down by your sides, palms flat on the ground, maybe a little under your hips. Reach your legs straight up creating a 90 degree angle at your hips and flex your feet. Keeping your legs straight and engaged, inhale to drop your right heel down towards the ground without touching, then exhale to pull your right leg back to 90 degrees. Repeat on the left. Alternate legs and don't let your lower back lift off the floor.

- Tricep Dips - 15-25 Reps

Sitting on a bench, a dining or folding chair or some secure seat, grip the edges of your seat with both hands at either side of you. Engage your abdominals and straighten your spine. Slide your hips forward off the seat, walking your feet a step or two forward, with your knees bent at a 90 degree angle. Keep your arms straight, torso upright and drop your shoulders away from your ears. Inhale to bend your elbows behind you to a 90 degree angle, lowering your body towards the floor. Exhale and push through your palms to straighten your arms. Repeat.

- Side Touches - 15-60 Seconds

Stand evenly between two feet, a little wider than hip distance apart, hands at your chest. Bend your legs at the knees and reach your hips back. Staying low, take a step to the right and reach your right hand down towards the floor on your right side (you don't have to be able to reach it, just reach for it) while counterbalancing by stretching your left toes to the left. Then again staying low, step on your left foot and reach your left hand towards the floor on your left while stretching through the right toes. Keep alternating side to side, set a tempo and keep it til you reach your time goal

- Knee Ups - 15-60 Seconds

Stand evenly between two feet, hip distance apart, hands in fists next to each other out in front of you, elbows at 90 degrees. Lift your right knee up to touch your fists, step back down on your right foot to lift your left knee to your fists. Repeat, alternating knees and picking the tempo, maybe even jumping, until your time goal.

· Booty Kickers - 15-60 Seconds

Continue your tempo from your Knee Ups, simply change your leg motion to pulling each foot to kick your glutes behind you and let the arms swing by your sides like you are running. Continue, alternating feet until your time goal.

Body Weight 4

· High Knee Skips - 15-60 Seconds

Stand evenly between two feet, hip distance apart, arms down by your sides. Keeping your left leg straight, push your right leg off the floor shooting your right knee high towards your chest. Put your right foot down immediately and repeat on the other side, pushing your left foot off the ground, shooting your left knee high towards your chest, then setting the foot down again. Repeat, alternating high knees and adding a skip into the rhythm. Set a tempo and keep it til your time goal.

· Half Burpees - 15-25 Reps

Start in your plank position, arms straight under your shoulders and feet shoulders width apart. Press your hands into the ground and keep them there as you exhale and hop or step your feet up to your hands, bending in the knees and aiming your feet outside your hands if you have to. Keeping your body weight in your hands, inhale to hop or step back to your plank position again. Repeat.

- Push Ups - 15-25 Reps

Start on the floor into your push up position, either on your toes or on your knees. Place a towel or yoga mat under your knees for support if needed. You can also do these standing by leaning at an angle against a wall, a counter or the back of a couch.

Place your hands at least shoulders width apart, maybe wider. Pull your belly button in towards your spine. Inhale to bend at the elbows lowering your body down almost to the floor, then exhale and push back up to your starting position. Repeat.

There are hundreds of ways to do a Push Up. Do what feels available to your body. If it hurts in a bad way, change something. Keep going!!

- Seated Russian Twist - 15-25 Each Side

Sit on a mat, towel or the floor and bend your knees in front of you, feet on the floor and legs together. Lift your legs up off the ground together any amount and balance on your sit bones. Pull your belly button to your spine, squeeze your thighs together to stabilize you and stretch your torso long. Clasp your hands together in front of you and twist your body to the right, reaching your fists towards the floor on that side (you don't have to touch it, just reach for it). Then twist to the left reaching your fists to the floor on the left. Repeat, exhaling as you twist, alternating sides.

• Hip Presses - 15-25 Reps

Lay on your back with your knees bent, feet flat on the floor and your arms by your sides, palms down. Legs can be touching or not, your call. Inhale to push your heels into the ground and engage your leg muscles to push your hips up to a straight line with your upper body. Exhale and lower your hips back down. Repeat.

• Walking High Knee Lunges - 10-15 Each Leg

Stand evenly between two feet, hip distance apart, hands on your waist. Inhale, taking an exaggerated step forward, rolling through your foot to plant it solidly beneath your leg. Then bend both knees equally to lower into a 90 degree lunge. Keep your forward knee over the ankle and your back knee from touching the ground. Exhale to shift your weight forward onto that front foot as you bring your back knee up to your chest, standing up straight. Then take an exaggerated step forward again with your raised foot, bending both knees low into a 90 degree lunge again. Walk forward and backward as much as you can until completing all your reps.

• Shoulder Flys - 15-25 Reps

Stand evenly between two feet, hip distance apart, arms straight down your sides. Drop your shoulders down away from your ears and wrap your shoulder blades around to hug your rib cage. Exhale and reach your fingers out wide to your sides, lifting your arms out to shoulder height, resisting like you have weight in your hands. Inhale to lower your arms back down to your sides, resisting like you are pushing through thick honey. Repeat.

12

Resistance Bands

If you want to add a little oomph to your workouts, or up the tension a bit, or get your heart beating a little more resistance bands are an easy and effective way to do that! Resistance bands challenge your muscles in different ways and can change your results quite a bit with consistency. They create more resistance the further you pull them, making them utterly adjustable. There are usually two shapes of bands you will find, long strips and round circles. Both have their benefits! I've included workouts utilizing each. Workout bands can be found in most sporting goods and fitness stores and sections in common retail chain stores. They shouldn't be too expensive at all. You can also tie a ripped pair of tights into a pretty good resistance band, so don't feel limited. I usually try most exercises with my middleweight band to start and adjust accordingly from there. Remember you can do any of these circuits 1-3 times through.

Let's get moving!

Long Strap Band Series 1

• Alternating Bicep Curls - 10-15 Each Arm

Stand on the band with your feet hip distance apart, holding an end in each hand, keeping your arms straight by your side with your palms facing forward. Keeping your elbows tucked into your sides, exhale and bend one elbow, lifting one fist at a time toward your shoulder. Inhale lowering your arm back down. Repeat, alternating sides.

• Tricep Extensions - 10-15 Each Arm

Stand with your left foot slightly in front of your right and step your right foot on the end of your resistance band. Hold the other end in your right hand and extend your arm straight over your head. Rest your left hand on your hip.Keeping your elbow close to the side of your head, inhale and lower your right forearm behind the back of your head until your elbow is bent at a 90 degree angle. Exhale to press your arm back straight overhead. Finish your reps, switch sides and repeat with the left arm.

• Squats - 15-25 Reps

Stand on your resistance band with your feet hips distance apart, holding an end of the band in each hand. Raise your hands close to your shoulders. Inhale as you bend your knees and shoot your hips back behind you, torso upright and abdominals engaged. Exhale to rise back up to standing. Repeat.

• Chest Fly - 15-25 Reps

Stand evenly between two feet, hip distance apart and run your resistance band across the back of your shoulders, holding an end in each hand and keeping your arms slightly bent. Keep your shoulders steady by dropping them away from your ears, exhale as you pull the ends toward the front of your body until your hands meet in front of your chest, keeping your arms strong and your elbows slightly bent. Inhale to release your arms back open. Repeat.

• Leg Extensions - 10-15 Each Leg

Stand evenly between two feet, hips distance apart. Wrap the band once around your right ankle and then step on both ends of the band with your left foot. Stand up straight with your hands on your hips or clasped in front of you. Exhale and extend your right leg straight out to the side, then inhale as you return it back down. Finish your reps for each side, then switch and repeat on the other side.

• Back Fly - 15-25 Reps

Stand evenly between two feet, hips distance apart and arms by your sides. Pull your belly button in and lean forward with a straight back, about 45 degrees. Let your arms hang down towards the ground. Shorten up the band in between your hands until there is no slack. Drop your shoulders down your spine, reach your arms long with a slight bend at the elbow. Keeping your arms long, exhale as you pull your arms open, pinching your shoulder blades together. Inhale to release the arms down. Repeat.

• Twisting Walking Lunges - 10-15 Each leg

Stand evenly between two feet, hips distance apart, arms out in front of you, wider than shoulders holding your band taught between your hands. Inhale, taking an exaggerated step forward, rolling through your foot to plant it solidly beneath your leg. Then bend both knees equally to lower into a 90 degree lunge. Keep your forward knee over the ankle and your back knee from touching the ground. As you bend your knees gently twist your spine towards your forward leg keeping the tension in the band. Exhale to press your front foot off the ground, pushing back to standing as your torso and arms swing to face forward. Repeat, alternating sides.

Long Strap Band Series 2

• Twisting Press Squats – 15–25 Reps

Stand on your resistance band with your feet hips distance apart, holding your bands loose in your hands. Lift your hands to your shoulders leading the bands behind your back so they are taught. Inhale as you bend your knees and shoot your hips back behind you, knees over ankles, torso upright and abdominals engaged. Exhale standing back up as you twist your torso to the right, pressing both hands up over your head. Inhale to bend your knees again, lowering into your squat, torso facing forward and hands back to your shoulders. Exhale to stand and twist to the left pressing your hands over head. Repeat as you alternate sides.

• Hip Extensions – 15–25 Reps

Stay standing on your resistance band, feet hips distance apart. Drop your arms down by your sides and shorten your grip on your band so it's tight. Inhale to bend your knees 45 degrees, shooting your hips back behind you and leaning forward 45 degrees. Exhale to straighten your legs, engaging the backs of your thighs to pull your chest upright. Repeat.

• Standing Tricep Kickbacks – 15-25 Reps

Keep standing on your resistance band. Pull your belly button in and lean forward with a straight back, about 45 degrees. Let your arms hang down towards the ground, shortening up your grip on your bands so there is no slack. Keeping your elbows close in towards your body, exhale and bend your elbows, pulling your fists to your ribs. Inhale to release your fists back towards the ground. Pull your belly button to your spine again and repeat.

• Hammer Curls – 10-15 Each Arm

Still standing on the band, drop your arms straight down by your sides with your thumbs facing forward, holding an end of the band in each hand so there is no slack. Keeping your elbows tucked into your sides, exhale and bend your right elbow lifting your fist to your shoulder. Inhale to lower your arm back down. Repeat, alternating sides.

• Stepping Lunges – 10-15 Each Leg

Stand evenly between two feet, hips distance apart and loop your band under your right foot, pull the band tight holding the ends in your fists. Inhale taking an exaggerated step backward, plant your foot solidly behind you. Then bend both knees equally to lower into a 90 degree lunge. Keep your forward knee over the ankle and your back knee from touching the ground. Exhale to press your back foot off the ground, pushing forward to stand. Finish your reps, switch sides and repeat with the left leg forward.

• Alternating Shoulder Raises - 10-15 Each Arm

Keeping your band looped under your left foot, stand evenly between two feet, hips distance apart holding your bands taught, arms straight down your sides. Drop your shoulders down away from your ears and wrap your shoulder blades around to hug your rib cage. Exhale and lift your right arm straight out to your side up to shoulder height. Inhale and release your arm back down to your side. Repeat lifting your left arm straight out and up to your side as you exhale and releasing your arm back down to your side as you inhale. Alternate until your complete your rep goal.

• Single Arm Wide Tricep Press - 10-15 Each Arm

Stand with your left foot slightly in front of your right and step your right foot on the end of your resistance band. Hold the other end in your left hand and extend your arm straight over your head. Rest your right hand on your hip. Keeping your elbow angled out to the side, inhale and lower your right forearm behind the back of your head until your elbow is bent at a 90 degree angle. Exhale to press your arm back straight overhead again. Finish your reps, switch sides and repeat with the right arm, stepping your left foot back on your band behind you.

• Chest Press - 15-25 Reps

Stand evenly between two feet, hip distance apart and run your resistance band across your back under your armpits, pulling the ends of the band to max tension straight forward in front of you at shoulder height. Inhale as you release your elbows back behind you, parallel to the ground in the shape of a W. Exhale to press your fists back forward and straighten your arms. Repeat.

Round Circular Band Series

- Resistance Squats – 15-25 Reps

Stand evenly between two feet, hip distance apart. Settle your loop band around your lower thighs, above your knees, so it's taught. Inhale as you bend both knees and reach your hips back behind you, keeping your knees over your toes as you lower down, creating a 90 degree angle with your legs. At the same time your arms bend at the elbow, bringing your hands either to your chest or straight out in front of you (or hold onto the couch for support). Exhale and press through your feet, engaging your leg muscles to stand up and drop your hands back down by your sides. Repeat.

- Leg Lifts, Forward, Side and Back – 10-15 Each Leg

Stand evenly between two feet, hips distance apart. Settle your loop band around your ankles so it's taught. Stand up straight with your hands on your hips or clasped in front of you. Exhale and extend your right leg straight out to the side, then inhale as you return it back down. Finish your reps for each side, then switch and repeat on the other side.

- Shoulder Presses – 15-25 Reps

Stand comfortably between two feet, arms stretched horizontally out in front of you, shoulder's width, palms facing in with your loop band taught around the back of your hands. Roll your shoulders down your spine. Exhale to pull your arms open a few inches. Inhale to release your arms back to shoulder's width. Repeat.

- Side to Side Steps – 15-25 Each Side

Stand evenly between two feet, hip distance apart. Settle your loop band around your lower thighs, above your knees, so it's taught. Bend both knees and reach your hips back behind you, keeping your knees over your toes as you lower down, creating a 45 degree angle with your legs. Bend your elbows, clasping your hands together in front of you. Maintaining this position, step wide to the right with your right foot then follow with your left, then step wide again with your right and follow with your left. Repeat to the otherside, stepping wide to the left with your left foot then following with your right, then step wide again with your left and follow with your right. Repeat, alternating sides.

- Step Lunges – 15-25 Each Side

Stand evenly between two feet, hips distance apart and loop your band around your lower thighs, above your knees, so it's taught. Inhale taking a step backward, plant your foot solidly behind you. Then bend both knees equally to lower into a 90 degree lunge. Keep your forward knee over the ankle and your back knee from touching the ground. Exhale to press your back foot off the ground, pushing forward to stand, maintaining the tension in your band the entire time. Repeat, alternating sides.

- Seated Rows - 15-25 Reps

Sit on a mat, towel or the floor and extend your legs together out in front of you. Sitting up tall, loop your band around your flexed feet and hold the other end in your hands, palms facing down. Keeping your elbows close in towards your body, exhale and bend your elbows, pulling your fists into your ribs. Inhale to release your fists back out in front of you. Repeat.

- Russian Twists - 15-25 Each Side

Still seated on the ground, move your loop band around your lower thighs, above your knees. Bend your knees and press them out until the band is taught. Lift your legs up off the ground any amount and balance on your sit bones. Pull your belly button to your spine, squeeze your thighs together to stabilize you and stretch your torso long. Clasp your hands together in front of you and twist your body to the right, reaching your fists towards the floor on that side (you don't have to touch it, just reach for it). Then twist to the left reaching your fists to the floor on the left. Repeat, exhaling as you twist, alternating sides.

13

Yoga

Yoga means to 'yoke' or join the movement of our body with the rhythm of our breath and the focus of our mind. That's what makes yoga the perfect 10 minute workout! For this entire book we are learning to be present while we move. Yoga does exactly this by inviting us to pay attention to the moment and breathe through our motions. Follow any of these sequences to get moving and feel better! Remember you can do any of these flows 1-3 times through.

Sun Salutation

• Tadasana - Mountain Pose

Stand evenly between two feet, hips distance apart, rooting all four corners of your feet to the ground. Stand tall, drop your shoulders down your spine. Breathe evenly as you bring your hands into prayer position.

- Urdhva Hastasana - Upward Salute

Inhale and raise your hands above your head into an upward salute with pinky fingers in and palms facing each other, slightly lifting your heart towards your hands, eyes gazing up.

- Uttanasana - Standing Forward Fold

Exhale folding forward at the waist, swan diving your arms as you reach for the ground or your shins. Let your knees bend slightly if needed.

- Ardha Uttanasana - Half-Standing Forward Fold

Inhale and lift halfway up, reaching your torso long, flattening your spine and engaging your abdominals. Stay looking down and bring your hands to your shins or upper thighs.

- Chaturanga Dandasana - Plank Pose

Exhale as you drop your hands to the mat under your shoulders and step back to your plank pose. Finish your exhale as you lower down to the ground, either in one piece on your toes or by dropping your knees then lowering your torso to the floor.

- Urdhva Mukha Svanasana - Upward Facing Dog

Inhale and press into your hands to extend your chest forward. Drop your shoulders back and down, arching your chest up, looking in front of you.

- Adho Mukha Svanasana - Downward Facing Dog

Exhale and lift your hips up and back pulling yourself into a triangle position. Reach your heels into the mat, they may not touch the ground, let your head hang loose, and press the ground firmly away from you, dropping your shoulder blades up the back and wrapping them around the rib cage.

Take 5 full breaths here, balancing the effort of the pose and relaxing into it and letting your body support you.

· Transition

Inhale to bend your knees and gaze between your hands. Exhale to step, walk or jump your feet back up to your hands, hips width apart, folding forward with an easy bend in your knees.

· Ardha Uttanasana - Half-Standing Forward Fold

Inhale and lift halfway up, reaching your torso long, flattening your spine and engaging your abdominals. Stay looking down and bring your hands to your shins or upper thighs.

· Uttanasana - Standing Forward Fold

Exhale folding forward at the waist, swan diving your arms as you reach for the ground or your shins. Let your knees bend slightly if needed.

· Urdhva Hastasana - Upward Salute

Inhale and raise your hands above your head into an upward salute with pinky fingers in and palms touching each other, slightly lifting your heart towards your hands, eyes gazing up.

- Tadasana – Mountain Pose

Exhale bringing your hands down in front of your chest. Stand tall and drop your shoulders down your spine.

Moon Salutation

- Urdhva Hastasana – Upward Salute

Inhale and raise your hands above your head into an upward salute with pinky fingers in and palms touching each other, slightly lifting your heart towards your hands, eyes gazing up. Pull your belly button to your spine.

- Standing Crescent Pose

Planting your left foot deep in the ground, bend to the right, reaching your fingertips long and arching through your left torso.
   Inhale back to center.
   Exhale to repeat to the left and inhale back to center.

- Goddess Pose

Exhale, stepping your feet out wide, toes turned out, torso long and upright and bending your knees and elbows to 90 degree angles, arms open to a cactus position.

- Trikonasana - Triangle Pose

Inhale to turn both feet to the right, left toes facing forward and right toes facing the side, reaching your arms straight out to your sides.

Exhale and hinge sideways at your hip to the right, reaching your fingertips away from each other and pulling your left hip away from the top of your head.

Inhale to plant your right hand on the ground, a block or your shin and rotate your spine open to the left, keeping your belly button engaged to your spine.

- Parsvottanasana - Pyramid Pose

Exhale and rotate your left arm down to your shin or the floor framing your right foot or leg, rotating your back foot more and squaring your hips and torso to face the floor, folding over your right leg.

- Lunge

Inhale stepping your left foot back behind you, leg straight while bending your right knee to a 90 degree angle. Reach your head away from your heels as you lift your thigh away from the ground.

- Skandasana - Side Legged Extended Squat

Exhale rotating your hips down to the ground in a half squat as your left knee and toes rotate to face the ceiling. Deepen into your bent right knee as your chest straightens up, palms meeting in front of your chest.

- Goddess Pose

Inhale, pressing through your right foot to push back to your wide center deep squat, toes turned out, torso upright, knees and elbows bent to 90 degree angles, arms open to a cactus position.

• Skandasana - Wide Legged Squat

Exhale dropping your hips down to your left heel in a half squat as your right leg straightens, knee and toes facing the ceiling. Torso is lifted up, palms meeting in front of your chest.

• Lunge

Inhale, rotating your hips to the ground, bending your left knee to a 90 degree angle and framing your left foot with both hands on the floor. Stretch your right leg straight behind you, toes down in a lunge.

• Parsvottanasana - Pyramid Pose

Exhale, lift your hips to the sky, straightening your left leg and pulling your right foot closer in, folding over your left leg.

• Trikonasana - Triangle Pose

Inhale to turn your right toes forward, planting your left hand on the ground, a block or your shin and stretching your torso long.
   Exhale rotating your right arm and torso open to the right, keeping your belly button engaged to your spine.

• Goddess Pose

Inhale, stepping your right foot out wide to the right side agian, dropping your hips low to your center deep squat, toes turned out, torso center and upright, knees and elbows bent to 90 degree angles, arms open to a cactus position.

- Urdhva Hastasana - Upward Salute

Inhale and step your feet in to standing, raise your hands above your head into an upward salute with pinky fingers in and palms touching each other, slightly lifting your heart towards your hands, eyes gazing up. Pull your belly button to your spine.

Exhale to bend to the left and repeat the sequence on the other side.

Vinyasa Flow

- Tadasana - Mountain Pose

Stand evenly between two feet, hips distance apart, rooting all four corners of your feet to the ground. Stand tall, drop your shoulders down your spine. Breathe evenly as you bring your hands into prayer position.

- Urdhva Hastasana - Upward Salute

Inhale and raise your hands above your head into an upward salute with pinky fingers in and palms facing each other, slightly lifting your heart towards your hands, eyes gazing up.

- Uttanasana - Standing Forward Fold

Exhale folding forward at the waist, swan diving your arms as you reach for the ground or your shins. Let your knees bend slightly if needed.

- Ardha Uttanasana - Half-Standing Forward Fold

Inhale and lift halfway up, reaching your torso long, flattening your spine and engaging your abdominals. Stay looking down and bring your hands to your shins or upper thighs.

- Chaturanga Dandasana - Plank Pose

Exhale as you drop your hands to the mat under your shoulders and step back to your plank pose. Finish your exhale as you lower down to the ground, either in one piece on your toes or by dropping your knees then lowering your torso to the floor.

- Urdhva Mukha Svanasana - Upward Facing Dog

Inhale and press into your hands to extend your chest forward. Drop your shoulders back and down, arching your chest up, looking in front of you.

- Adho Mukha Svanasana - Downward Facing Dog

Exhale and lift your hips up and back pulling yourself into a triangle position. Reach your heels into the mat, they may not touch the ground, let your head hang loose, and press the ground firmly away from you, dropping your shoulder blades up the back and wrapping them around the rib cage.

• Utthita Adho Mukha Svanasana - Extended Downward Facing Dog

Inhale reaching your right leg straight up strong behind you.

Exhale bringing the right foot back down, bending your knee to your chest and planting your right foot between your hands in a low lunge, adjusting your back foot as necessary.

• Virabhadrasana 1 - Warrior 1

Leaving your hips where they are, inhale your arms forward and up over head, shoulders wide and palms facing in, lifting your torso tall. Right leg is at a 90 degree angle, back leg is straight and strong

• Virabhadrasana 2 - Warrior 2

Again leaving the hips at the same height they are, exhale to rotate your left hip open and your left heel to the ground, windmilling your left arm back parallel to your left leg and dropping your right arm horizontal over your right thigh at shoulder level. Reach your fingers away from each other.

• Parsa Virabhadrasana - Reverse Warrior

Leave your lower half where it is, inhale and hinge to the left at your waist, drawing your left fingers down your thigh and reaching your right arm arching over your torso.

• Utthita Parsvakonasana - Extended Side Angle

Exhale to windmill your right fingers back up, over and down the ground by your right foot, deepening into your right side lunge as the left arm follows reaching over your torso extending over your right knee.

• Virabhadrasana 2 - Warrior 2

Remaining in your deep lunge as much as possible, inhale to windmill your left arm back up and over to your left side, pulling your torso straight up, belly button to spine and right arm extended horizontally over your bent right knee.

• Chaturanga Dandasana - Plank Pose

Exhale as you windmill your hands the other direction to the mat under your shoulders and step back to your plank pose. Finish your exhale as you lower down to the ground, either in one piece on your toes or by dropping your knees then lowering your torso to the floor.

• Urdhva Mukha Svanasana - Upward Facing Dog

Inhale and press into your hands to extend your chest forward. Drop your shoulders back and down, arching your chest up, looking in front of you.

• Adho Mukha Svanasana - Downward Facing Dog

Exhale and lift your hips up and back pulling yourself into a triangle position. Reach your heels into the mat, they may not touch the ground, let your head hang loose, and press the ground firmly away from you, dropping your shoulder blades up the back and wrapping them around the rib cage.

- Repeat steps 8 – 16 for the left side. Alternate sides 1–3 times through, evenly.

- Transition

Inhale to bend your knees and gaze between your hands. Exhale to step, walk or jump your feet back up to your hands, hips width apart, folding forward with an easy bend in your knees.

- Ardha Uttanasana – Half-Standing Forward Fold

Inhale and lift halfway up, reaching your torso long, flattening your spine and engaging your abdominals. Stay looking down and bring your hands to your shins or upper thighs.

- Uttanasana – Standing Forward Fold

Exhale folding forward at the waist, swan diving your arms as you reach for the ground or your shins. Let your knees bend slightly if needed.

- Urdhva Hastasana – Upward Salute

Inhale and raise your hands above your head into an upward salute with pinky fingers in and palms touching each other, slightly lifting your heart towards your hands, eyes gazing up.

- Tadasana – Mountain Pose

Exhale bringing your hands down in front of your chest. Stand tall and drop your shoulders down your spine.

14

The Cool Downs

You did it! You made a positive investment in your overall health and wellness and moved your body today. Congratulations!!

We end any movement session with a few minutes of cooling down for a few reasons. We want to ease our heart rates back down to our resting rate, as well as let our blood pressure lower naturally. By easing our bodies down we prevent potential injuries as our muscles, tendons and ligaments as they get to release slowly back to their resting states too. We also prevent any light headedness or dizziness, preventing fainting. Light movements help move lactic acid out of our muscles easing recovery time and intensity too. Just like warming up you only need 3-5 minutes of easy, gentle movement.

One and Done Cool Downs

1. Easy Jog
2. Brisk Walk
3. Arm Swings
4. Gentle Stretching
5. Spinal Twist
6. Gentle Somatic Body Shaking

Easy Cool Down Stretches

- Quads

Stand easily between your feet, shift your weight to your left foot. Bend your right knee bringing your right foot up to your hips behind. Grab your right foot and hold, stretching the front of your right thigh. Drop your right foot, shift your weight to your right and repeat with your left foot bent up behind you.

- Shoulders

Both feet on the ground, standing easily, cross your straight right arm over your chest. Use your left arm to stretch your right arm further across your body. Release and repeat for your left arm.

- Triceps

Swing your right arm up and behind your head, bending at the elbow.

Reach your left hand up to your right elbow and use the weight of your left arm to stretch your right triceps. Release and repeat for your left arm.

- Sides

Swing your right arm up over head and reach for the wall to your left. Stretch your right ribs open as you breathe. Release and repeat for your left arm.

- Chest

Clasp your hands behind your back and either pull your fists down to the ground, lift your heart forward and up, or both.

- Glutes

From standing, shift your weight to your left and cross your right ankle over your left lower thigh, above your knee, in a figure 4 shape. Clasp your hands in front of you and squat low until you feel the stretch. Release and repeat for your left glutes.

- Hips

Sit down and bend both knees, opening them wide bringing the bottoms of your feet together. Hold your feet as you press them down into the ground, pressing your knees open as well.

- Hamstrings and Calves

Extend both your legs straight forward in front of you. Bend your right knee, letting it fall open to the side as you bring the bottom of your right foot to your inner left thigh. Inhale to sit up straight and square your torso to your straight leg, then exhale and fold softly forward. Breathe, release and repeat on the other side.

- Side Glutes

Extend both your legs straight forward in front of you. Bend your right knee, this time keep the knee up towards the ceiling and cross your right foot over your left leg. Inhale to sit up straight, then exhale to twist towards your right leg using your arms to help and stabilize you. Breathe, release and repeat on the other side.

- Abs

Lie face down on your mat or the floor and place your palms beneath your shoulders. As much or as little as you desire, press through your hands to lift your chest and stretch the front of your body. Breathe and release when ready.

- Back

Shift your hips back to your heels, settling your weight on your legs, opening your knees wide so your chest can fall between them. Arms either still extended forward or wrapped down your sides, extend your forehead to the ground and breathe.

Sit up slowly when you are done.

15

Conclusion

There you have it! Everything you need to get up off the couch and get moving! No matter where your fitness journey goes, remember that taking small steps add up, simple actions get us up and moving and understand that doing just a little every day is better than nothing. Keep things straightforward and simple... just Move!!

Thank you for joining me! I hope you had as much fun working through this book as I had writing it. If you found this book helpful in any way I would be deeply appreciative if you left a favorable review for the book on Amazon!